Intermittent Fasting

A Beginner's Guide To Losing Body Fat With Intermittent Fasting (21 Day Ritual)

Table of Contents

Introduction

I want to thank you for choosing this book, '*Intermittent fasting - A beginner's guide to losing body fat with intermittent fasting (21 day ritual).*'

It is no secret that weight loss is hard to achieve. We have been fed stories right from a young age that having a healthy body comes from eating three healthy meals a day. Almost everyone follows this theory and tends to blindly follow a routine that incorporates a breakfast, lunch and dinner.

We have all heard from our elders that we should start our days with a heavy and filling breakfast, a medium light lunch and a very light dinner. It is what they say has worked best for them. However, we no longer lead the same kind of lives and will require a change to our diet in order to suit our current needs. This is not the only popular theory doing the rounds, as there are others similar. One well-known theory is to split your three regular meals into 5 or 6 smaller ones so that your level of metabolism stays high. But no one really knows whether this is good advice or if it will work for all.

Well, to break away from these theories and to start something completely opposite, you can give Intermittent Fasting a try. Intermittent fasting refers to a weight loss plan where you are not told what to eat rather when to eat. You will be taken through a set of fasting plans where you will not be made to eat several meals and achieve weight loss and gain vitality by controlling meal times.

This book will serve as your ultimate guide to intermittent fasting and teach you how exactly you can incorporate it into your life. It will serve as an inspiration to all those who have tried everything and still not found the answer. Not only will you be able to get rid of excess weight but also maintain a stable body weight. Do not worry if you happen to be someone who tends to gain weight right after going off a diet. The intermittent fast is designed to keep weight off for good. It is a lifestyle choice and will not leave you with the side effects associated with other diets.

Stop blaming things today and get started with an intermittent fast! It will not be long before you start seeing positive effects. You will be surprised to notice that the fat is being automatically gobbled up just by moving your meal timings. So, stop wasting your time going through other diet-based books that promise you things that will never happen in reality. It would be foolish to think you can shed excess weight just by eating foods that can cut down on your weight. Instead, go for something that is time tested and sure to leave you with positive benefits.

This book was written after studying the diet and taking it up for at least a year. The advice is genuine and is bound to help you feel lighter and better. Just by following the advice given, you are sure to take up the diet on a serious note and do yourself a favor.

It is obvious that you will find it a little difficult at the beginning but you will get better at it as and when you take on the diet. You will begin to realize that you alone can bring about a difference and allow the fast to modify your body. There should no longer be a blame game and you have to take matters into your own hands.

You will be able to do things you were never able to do before and be in a great position to take up physical tasks that you thought were beyond you.

The intermittent fast will allow you to strike a balance between your weight loss goals and your desire to attain excellent health. It will be much simpler than taking on a traditional diet and require less effort from you. Once you have started, you have to do very little in terms of maintaining it. You will pretty much go onto autopilot and the diet will let you lose weight rapidly. It will boost your digestion and metabolism and put you on the right track to develop the body of your dreams.

I'm sure you are now extremely curious to know more about the diet and take it up to full throttle.

So without any further delay, let us begin!

Chapter One: What Is Intermittent Fasting?

The very first thing you have to know about intermittent fasting is that it is not a diet! It can be viewed as a lifestyle choice that you make to eliminate a few meals and snacks per day. But do not confuse it with starvation, as you have to eat to provide your body with enough energy and nutrients to keep you going.

The intermittent fast is a simple concept where you alternate between periods of eating and fasting. It is a matter of knowing when to eat as opposed to what to eat. It calls for the consumption of everyday calories within a certain period of time and remaining in fasting phase for the rest of the day.

Here are some of the fasting plans to choose from.

The 16/8 fast

The 16/8 diet is one version where you fast for 16 hours and eat in the next 8 hours. It is a very simple plan. All you have to do is figure out a period when you would like to consume your normal three meals. Say, for example, you have your dinner by 8 p.m. The next meal has to be consumed only after 12 noon the next day. You will have to skip breakfast and go for lunch instead. It is your choice to have 3 meals or limit it to two, i.e., lunch, snack and dinner or lunch and dinner in the next 8 hours.

This intermittent fast is easier to adopt for those who are accustomed to skipping breakfast. All you have to do is ensure you do not consume anything in the fasting hours. You are, however, allowed to have liquids. You can have any type of liquid including juices, fruit infused water, coconut water, etc. Just make sure you keep a tab on the calorie level and avoid sugary drinks or those with calories.

The 5:2 fast

The 5:2 intermittent fast is a version that is designed to help you shed excess weight within a few months. It is one where you consume a regular diet for 5 days and fast on the remaining 2 days. These 2 days can be weekends or any two days of your choice. It is not advisable to go completely without food on these two days. Limit your calorie intake to 500 or 600. There are no restrictions as to what you can have for the remaining 5 days. Men should limit it to 600 and women should go for 500 calories on the fasting days.

Warrior diet

The warrior diet is a rather simple form of intermittent fast. It can be considered as a beginner's intermittent fast. All you have to do is go for small portions of vegetables and fruit in the mornings. You then have a regular meal at night. There is no restriction on what you can consume for dinner. The warrior diet is so called because athletes and sportsmen trying to get fit follow this plan.

Eat stop eat

The eat stop eat is a type of diet that is said to be on the extreme side. It calls for you to not eat anything for an entire day. This is only ideal if you are accustomed to fasting. If you are not, then you might end up sending your body into starvation mode. So, ensure that you only take up this diet if you are comfortable with the idea of not consuming a meal for 24 hours straight. Let's say you consume your meal at 2 p.m. The next has to be consumed at 2 p.m. the next day. There are no restrictions to what can be consumed the rest of the week.

Alternate fasting

This is an extension of the previous type of fast where you fast on alternate days. If you eat your regular three meals on Sunday then you fast on Monday, eat again on Tuesday and fast on Wednesday and so on. Keep alternating between fasting and eating. This can be quite taxing and should be followed by those who are prepared for it. You can always consume liquids on fasting days. They have to be controlled in terms of calorie intake. It is best to go for this diet during the last few stages of weight loss. Start with the 16/8 and then go for the 5:2 before going for the eat stop eat version and then gradually take on alternate fasting.

The choice is yours. Choose any of these fasting types to get started with intermittent fasting. Here are some tips to help you.

- Make sure you choose the correct time frame to have your meals and stick to it. The idea behind the intermittent fast is that you try and reduce the number of meals you consume per day. Most of us are accustomed to consuming three meals a day with 2 or 3 snacks thrown in between. The intermittent fast aims at reducing the number of meals consumed to 2 meals per day.

- The idea is to go from an 8-hour eating window to 6-hour window and finally to a 4-hour window.
- The best way to go about this is by first taking on the 8-hour eating window and cutting out the morning snack. This snack is usually consumed between breakfast and lunch. Most of us start feeling peckish at around the 12 noon mark and reach for something to munch on. Having this snack can not only make you delay your lunch, it can also make you go back on your fast. So, a good idea would be to consume a heavy breakfast. Eat at least 450 calories and include an egg omelette with an avocado shake. For lunch, go for 450 calories and have chicken curry with flatbread. For dinner, go for something light such as a vegetable salad and a glass of fresh juice.
- The next challenge would be to cut out the evening snack. According to research, those who consume a late evening or late-night snack end up gaining weight much more easily. Make sure you do not dig into a snack before dinner. Start your day with the same menu as mentioned in the previous point. Consume a heavier lunch of about 500 calories. Keep dinner simple and limit it to 400 calories.
- By following the previous two steps, you will have successfully gone from 5 meals a day to 3 by cutting out two snacks. The next step would be to cut out one of the meals.
- It might sound like you are being asked not to eat anything at all. But it is not the case as you can pack in the same number of calories within two meals. The meal you wish to drop depends on you. Some prefer to do away with breakfast while some prefer to skip lunch and others forgo dinner. Since you know your body best, it is entirely up to you to choose which two meals to go for.
- Once you have decided on the meals, the next step is to start narrowing down the eating window. If you are used to eating at 12 noon followed by lunch at 4 p.m. and dinner by 8 p.m., then eliminate lunch and go for heavier breakfast and dinner.
- Next, close the gap between the two by having lunch at 1 p.m. and dinner at 7 p.m. This will bring down the eating window to 6 hours. Continue this for a couple of weeks.

- Next, reduce the eating window to 4-hours. Have your lunch by 2 p.m. and your dinner by 6 p.m. This can sound a bit daunting but taking it up can help you build a strong and healthy body. In fact, it can alter your thought process and make you a productive and happy person.
- Remember to have visual reminders everywhere. Paste your meal plan on the fridge door so that you are motivated to stick to it.
- Bear in mind that not all calories are the same. You have to know what to eat and what to avoid. Just because you are eating just two meals doesn't mean you go for junk and processed foods. These should never be an option. The calories should come by way of healthy foods. Don't worry about cutting down on a majority of the meals. You are not denying your body anything. You are only modifying the structure of meal consumption.
- Apart from meal consumption, you must also focus on sleeping well. The more you sleep, the more calories your body burns. When you sleep, your body automatically starts burning calories. If there are less calories to burn, then it will start drawing from your fat reserves. This means that you do not even have to exercise and that sleep alone will do the job for you.
- It is also very easy for you to take on the diet if you push your fasting periods to night times. When you sleep, you are less likely to crave food. You will also not feel like getting up and grabbing something to eat. This will make it easier for you to stick to the fast.
- Remember that it is always best to eat your last meal as early as possible. Think of consuming it by 5 p.m. if possible and sleep by 9 p.m. This will catapult your weight loss process.

Chapter Two: What to Eat While Intermittent Fasting

In the previous chapter, we looked at the basics of the intermittent fast and what you need to know in order to get started on it.

In this chapter, we will look at some of the foods that you simply must include in your diet while you take up the fast.

Water

This is definitely the most important element to consume when you take up the intermittent fast. Water can act as an elixir when it comes to losing weight. You must keep your body hydrated and ensure that all the toxins are dissolved and eliminated. All your organs need water to remain fresh and healthy; right from your liver to gut to digestive tract, water helps to keep these organs working smoothly. Drink at least 8 to 10 glasses of water a day and focus more on the fasting period. It is obvious that it will get a little monotonous and so, a good idea is to consume fruit infused water. This refers to water that has fruit and herbs infused into it. Fill up a jar with water and toss in fruit and herbs such as oranges, lemons, mint leaves and a dash of cinnamon. Consume this every few hours. Remember that the intermittent fast can be quite taxing at times and lead to side effects such as headache and nausea. In such a case, only water can help you out and put an end to these.

Fish

Fish can be considered as a miracle food as it can greatly help with weight loss. According to dietary guidelines, it is important for people to consume at least 6 to 8 ounces of fish every week. Fish contains a lot of nutrients. It is rich in fats and proteins. It is also rich in vitamin D. and this means you do not have to worry about denying your body these nutrients by taking on the fast. You do not have to reach for supplements if you are able to consume fish regularly. Fish is also rich in DHA, which helps in brain development. You will see that your mind is fresher and you are able to think better. Your productivity will increase and stress will be curbed.

Avocado

You might wonder why avocado is in this list considering it is one of the fattiest foods out there. However, you must understand that the fasting phase can take a toll on your body and so you must consume foods that can keep you going. Avocado is rich in monounsaturated fat, which is great for those who tend to get hungry quite fast. It keeps you feeling full for longer. You will not find yourself reaching out to eat a snack. Avocado is quite versatile and can be added to your breakfast or lunch menu. Those who tend to include it in their breakfast menu are generally able to go without food for longer periods of time without complaining about hunger.

Leafy greens

If there is one type of vegetable that we remember being told to consume by our parents then it has to be leafy green vegetables. As we know, leafy green vegetables are loaded with multiple nutrients that are great for your body. These include the likes of kale, broccoli, lettuce, etc. These are loaded with fiber. Fiber, as you know, keeps your body going when you suffer from digestive issues such as constipation. You are sure to go through it when you adopt the intermittent fast. In such a case, it becomes that much more important to consume these vegetables to keep your stomach in good shape. Fiber also makes you feel fuller and not feel too hungry between meals.

Potatoes

As mentioned earlier, the goal is to consume foods that are filling and can keep you going for hours, one such being potatoes. Potatoes are rich in carbs that can keep you sated for hours. Make sure you either steam and mash them or roast them without the addition of any oil or fat. Deep frying them is never an option. Try to consume them with their skin on as the skin contains a lot of nutrition.

Probiotics

When it comes to digestion, both your liver and gut play a very important role. Both of them need a healthy dose of probiotics in order to function optimally. If you have an unhealthy gut then you might suffer from side effects such as constipation and even leaky gut syndrome. The best way to combat these is by consuming as many probiotics as possible. Some natural foods rich in probiotics include kombucha and kefir. Add these to your meals and you are sure to experience positive benefits. An alternative is to go for probiotic supplements. Make sure you know which ones to go for. It would be best to consult a physician first.

Assorted berries

There is nothing better than consuming fresh berries in the mornings. They are loaded with antioxidants and vital nutrients required to keep your body healthy. Strawberries, raspberries, blueberries and gooseberries all are great for you. Just toss them into the blender with some milk or yogurt to make a smoothie. According to studies, those who consumed berries regularly were able to remain within their ideal body weight and did not gain too much weight over longer periods of time.

Eggs

An important aspect of losing weight is building lean muscles. Lean muscles replace regular ones and prevent fat from getting stored. The best way to build lean muscle is by consuming foods rich in proteins. One important source of proteins is eggs. Those who consume eggs for breakfast are in a better position to develop lean muscles and not go hungry before the next meal. Eggs can be quite versatile and cooked in any way you like. Hard-boil them the previous day so that you have a ready meal the next morning. Simply toss them in a pan to scramble them. It only takes a few minutes to cook them.

Whole grains

One aspect of maintaining a clean and healthy diet is going for whole grains. The intermittent fast promotes consumption of these, as they are easier for the body to digest and keep the system clean. They are also loaded with proteins and fiber. Do not limit yourself to the usual such as wheat and oats and go for something different such as Bulgar, amaranth and flax.

Legumes

If you wish to remain full for longer and not feel hungry or peckish too often then there is nothing better than legumes and beans. These cannot only be quite flavorful but also loaded with fiber. The body does not easily digest fiber. In fact, the body cannot digest it at all but makes extra effort in trying to digest it thereby drawing into the fat reserves. It is, therefore, best to load up on fiber in order to lose weight easily. There are many options to pick from including peas, lentils, green beans, fava, black-eyed peas, etc. These easily fit into soups and salads.

Nuts

Nuts are fatty no doubt, but they contain good fat. Not all fat is bad fat as there can be some good fat as well. Polyunsaturated fats are said to be good for the body and can keep you feeling full for longer. You will not feel hungry if you munch on some walnuts or almonds. But make sure you make them a part of your meal and do not snack on them. Snacking on them can leave you feeling full and disrupt your meal plan. Do not worry about the calorie aspect. Nuts are not as calorific as you may have thought. They contain far less calories than some of the other fatty foods that people tend to snack on.

These happen to be superfoods that you must include in your diet while you take up intermittent fasting.

Chapter Three: Foods to Avoid While Intermittent Fasting

Processed foods

Processed foods include the likes of biscuits, wafers, chips, cakes and sugary drinks such as cola. These will only add to your woes and counteract your weight loss goals. Try to avoid these at all costs. Do not hit the aisles at the supermarket that carry these foods. Remember to never go shopping on an empty stomach, as you will feel tempted to reach for a packet or snack.

Junk foods

Make it a point to cut out all junk food from your diet. There should be no room for burgers, pizzas and pastas that contain a lot of fat. It might be tempting to go for a cheat meal once in a while, but it is important not to do so as it can lead to a habit.

Alcohol

Although wine is said to be quite healthy, it would be best to limit it to just 1 serving per week. Try your best to avoid consuming hard liquor.

Although it is said that the intermittent fast does not tell you what not to eat, it is best to avoid these when you wish to lose weight.

Chapter Four: Intermittent Fasting and Weight Loss

Now that you have a basic idea of what the intermittent fast is all about and the superfoods to incorporate, it is time to look at how the fast can help with weight loss.

It is obvious that our bodies go through different reactions when we consume food and go on a fast. When a person eats, their body requires a little time to process the food and digest it. It does its best to burn away as much as it can. Once it is done, the remainder is stored as fat. The amount of fat depends on the type of meal you have eaten.

On the other hand, when you take up intermittent fasting, you put your body in a position where it readily draws from the available fat reserves. This makes it easier for you to lose excess weight and keep it from adding back on.

You can condition your body to think and act a certain way. It will be easier for your body to burn away whatever is available in the bloodstream. If you have had a sugary meal, then the body will have to put in a lot of effort to spend it all. It will not be able to do so unless you got on a treadmill for an hour just after the meal.

The body has to burn carbs to supply fuel to carry out daily activities. If you keep supplying your body with this energy then it will never resort to drawing it out from the fat reserves.

So, when you fast, you are denying your body any easy carbs to burn as fuel. This forces it to dig deep into the reserves and draw them out to burn as fuel. There will be no readily available glucose in your bloodstream, which makes it ideal for weight loss to set in. So, this burning fat results in weight loss.

Having said all that, do not expect to lose weight within a month. Although the process sounds quite simple, it can be a complicated process. Do not assume that you will start losing weight just by not eating food for a few hours. It requires systematic planning and execution. Intermittent fasting is not a fad or yo-yo diet. It is a lifestyle modification.

You might be a little taken aback by how slow it goes at the beginning. But you will be surprised at the level at which you will begin to lose fat and develop leaner muscle. You will actually feel your body shrinking and being able to get into smaller clothes. In fact, you will be able to show off your curves and contours and further boost your confidence to get into fasting on a more serious note.

Although the intermittent fast is designed to help you lose weight without indulging in physical exercise, it is always advisable to do some. Not only will it help you tone down more but also eliminate the melted fat in your body. The body will find it easier to draw from the reserves. All you have to do is provide enough energy to your body to carry out the exercises. There is plethora of choices when it comes to exercises. You can go for skipping, running, swimming, gymming, etc.

Insulin

I'm sure you have heard about insulin. Most people associate it with diabetes and how an insulin dysfunction can lead to it. When we consume food, our body automatically produces insulin. The faster your body is able to use this insulin, the better the results. This means that your body will be able to better break down the consumed food depending on how fast it absorbs the insulin and puts it to work. This can offset weight loss much faster and make you lose weight easily. In fact, it can lead to the creation of leaner muscle that will replace the fat cells.

When you fast, you increase insulin sensitivity. Your body becomes that much more sensitive to insulin release and absorption. This means that it goes after the existing glucose in your body that is stored as fat. It draws energy from this glucose to supply your body with fuel.

You have to acquaint yourself with the concept of glycogen. It refers to a starch that is present in your liver and muscles. Your body tends to turn to it in case it needs energy. However, in most cases it ends up being dissipated when you start fasting. If you are able to get your body to bring down its levels by working out regularly then it will further increase your insulin sensitivity.

This implies that physical activity automatically makes it easier for the body to draw from reserves and use it to up the insulin availability. Food that is stored as glycogen will be burned away to supply energy.

So, plan out your exercise regime in such a way that you take up a rigorous routine right after a heavy meal. Since you are most likely going to consume a heavy breakfast, it would be best to go for an exercise routine about 2 hours after breakfast. Keep it light and fun. If you go for a rigorous routine then you will end up losing interest in it, as it will be too taxing. Try out new workouts such as Zumba or go for belly dancing. Not only will you lose weight but also thoroughly enjoy yourself. Don't worry if you feel like you do not have the body or moves for it, you are not doing it to enter a competition.

Just make sure you have fun and do not think of it as an arduous task. It always helps to have company. Ask someone to join in so that it does not get too awkward and you remain motivated to persist with it. With time, you will realize that you are automatically getting better at it and can use it to your advantage.

Now imagine adopting this lifestyle and compare it with what you currently have. Weight loss is not easy and requires a lot of effort from your end. On a normal day you would have consumed 5 meals and had no exercise. It is obvious that your glycogen levels will be super high. These will not get used up at all and will get stored as fat. You have to give your body enough means to get rid of the fat reserves.

You might have noticed that most diabetic patients are overweight. This is because they will have a lot of glucose in their body that is not used up fully. This leads to insulin dysfunction. It is therefore important to be well within your ideal BMI and make sure you remain within your ideal weight range.

HGH

Apart from insulin, there is another hormone that is known to help induce weight loss and keep it off. Known as the human growth hormone or HGH, it is one that helps strengthen muscle power. As we know, muscles are very important and one must try to build lean muscle.

HGH helps to enhance exercise performance. Your body will be in a better position to fulfill exercise routines. Those who are obese tend to have lower levels of response to this hormone's stimuli. HGH aides to offset lipolysis, which refers to the breaking down of lipids or fat reserves in the body.

According to a study, obese people who were put on a diet and given HGH were able to increase their weight loss by almost double as compared to those who were not put on it. The best part of the experiment was that they were able to reduce visceral fat, which happens to be one of the toughest forms of fat to fight away. In the group that did not receive HGH, it was found that they had lost out on lean body mass. But with the group that received the hormones, their lean body mass had increased.

This shows that HGH is great when it comes to losing weight holistically. When you fast, this hormone automatically increases.

This hormone is consistently produced and secreted all through the day and night. You do not have to do anything, as the fast will take care of it.

HGH in combination with an increase in insulin sensitivity will end up making weight loss that much easier. Your body will be ready for lean muscle growth.

To put it simply, intermittent fasting tells your body the best way in which the food you consume can be used. It makes sure your body knows that the food is being supplied so that it can start the process of digging into the fat reserve and use it as fuel. This automatically offsets weight loss.

Treat every meal as a celebratory meal and enjoy it. Do not be in a hurry to eat something and rush to your next job. Make it a point to sit down and savor the meal. Spend at least 30 minutes understanding all the flavors involved, the textures involved, etc.

Chapter Five: How Intermittent Fast Differs from Other Diets

By now, you must have understood that the intermittent fast is unlike any fad diet. It does not tell you want to eat. It only tells you when to eat. Most diets will ask you to consume many meals per day instead of 2. Here is why they suggest this routine.

Most diets want you to believe that eating more is a measure to burn more calories. Since the body needs energy to burn off the food that is consumed, consuming more food provides more energy. So, if you break up your meals into smaller ones then your body is constantly burning calories. Although this sounds like the perfect plan to maintain your ideal body weight, it is definitely not a good one. It more or less takes the same number of calories to burn away your current calorie intake. So, you do not have to keep eating all the time to burn it away. So you will not get anything by eating 5 or 6 meals.

But if you were to ask someone who is following this routine then they would tell you that they are feeling fitter and better because they are eating smaller meals and the body has more time to digest it. However, that is not how it works and the body keeps adding it all up. So, in effect, you are only adding more and more to your weight woes.

Most people will not agree that they are better off with 2 meals instead of 5 or 6. It is how they are programmed to think. They will assume that it is easier to eat a little at a time and digest it. They will criticize 2 meals a day as forcing the body to go into starvation mode. This is not true. As discussed earlier, it is not important to focus on what you eat. You should know when exactly to eat the meal.

Now you might think that people who finish the fasting phase will lose control during the eating phase. There is a possibility to this, especially if the person is not accustomed to portion control. The key is to know exactly when to stop eating. Don't go on eating just because you think you have to load up on energy to last you through the fasting phase. Eat like you would a normal meal. The idea is to push your body into a state of fasting. So, it is obvious that you have to cut back on excessive eating during the eating phase. You have to learn to take control of the meal and not allow it to dictate over you.

So, if you have been following the 6-meal routine then it is better to rethink the strategy. Chances are high you are consuming more calories than recommended. This type of routine works best for those who are already thin and have a small stomach. They will not eat much anyway and thus their meals can be split up into smaller portions and consumed all through the day. They do so just to be able to remain energetic all the time. If you are fat then you need to cut down on your meals to supply the energy and not keep eating.

You will also end up affecting your rate of metabolism. Metabolism refers to the rate at which food is burned away. If you keep eating then you will not be able to burn it away easily. You have to build leaner muscle to keep the fat out. You must limit your meals to just two and take up regular exercises.

If you think about having too many meals then there are high chances you will settle for the wrong choice of food. It is easier to turn to junk and processed foods as compared to healthier options if you are asked to have many meals.

Paleo

The Paleo man walked on Earth thousands of years ago. He is said to have been quite healthy with a lean and strong frame and little to no lifestyle related illnesses such as stress and anxiety. One aspect of his diet involved fasting. It is obvious that there were no supermarkets back then where the Paleolithic man could pick up groceries. He ate whatever was available, whenever it was available. This meant going through periods of fasting. This helped them develop strong and lean bodies. It was almost impossible for them to develop obesity, as there was no access to junk and processed foods. They did not drink or smoke either thereby cutting out almost all the things that can lead to obesity.

The intermittent fast gives you the chance to mimic their food habits. You go through periods of fasting and then eat within a small window. This can do wonders for your body. A neat trick is to go for meals that use rare ingredients. For example, instead of going for regular wheat flour that is easily available at the supermarket, go for fox millet flour, which is quite hard to come by. This will make the meals more special and you will savor it more. You will also go through regular periods of fasting.

According to a recent study, it was found that it is not how much you eat that determines weight loss or gain but instead the quality of food you consume. So, make sure you make meals using the best of what is available to you. Make the effort to hit organic supermarkets to pick out foods that are healthy. You should love your meals. As mentioned several times already, the intermittent fast is not about forgoing a meal or skipping something just because you think it will help you shed a few extra pounds. It is about being able to eat whatever you like. Just make sure you follow the mealtime table and have the meal at the right time.

Experiment with new foods and flavors to cut out monotony. Go for different fruit and vegetables. Try to have at least 4 different colored vegetables on your plate during every meal.

It is all about modifying and customizing a meal to your liking. Do what works best for you and you are sure to see the best results.

As you can see, the intermittent fast is quite different from regular diets.

Chapter Six: Health Benefits of Intermittent Fasting

The intermittent fast provides a plethora of health benefits that are bound to leave you feeling like a new person. Here are some of them in detail.

Heart health

When it comes to maintaining a healthy body, you have to pay attention to all the vital organs. This includes your heart, brain, liver, gut and kidneys. They have to be in top shape in order for your body to remain healthy. You must pay attention to heart health right from a young age. You can do so by taking up intermittent fasting. The fast helps controlling LDL levels in your body. It takes care of blood pressure and ensures that your heart remains healthy. You will find it easier to take up tasks and not feel too tired at the end of the day.

Eating less

As you know, you tend to consume less meals on the diet. In fact, you bring it down to just 2 meals per day. Once you start doing that, your body automatically starts to process the consumed food better. The choice is yours to make and you can go for lunch and dinner or breakfast and lunch or breakfast and dinner etc. By consuming fewer meals you give your metabolism a boost. Once you get the hang of the diet, your metabolism will speed up and help you lose weight faster.

Healthier mind

It is no secret that the mind controls everything. It even controls your weight loss. If a person has an unhealthy mind then he is bound to pile on pounds. People like this will start consuming unhealthy foods and snacks. This will only add to their weight issues. An unhealthy mind also tends to attract stress and anxiety, which may add further to the negativity felt. The intermittent fast is designed to eliminate the consumption of all those foods that can create an abundance of cortisol in the brain. This chemical leads to stress. It promotes consumption of foods that release serotonin, which helps to combat stress and thereby keeps the mind fresh and open to accepting the positive results provided by the diet.

Better hormones

Hormones control a large portion of the functions that go on in your body. It is extremely important for your hormones to function optimally. A hormone known as HGH or human growth hormone helps control weight gain. It also promotes weight loss and is thus extremely important for your body. The intermittent fast helps release this hormone. This helps you lose weight faster and ensure that it is kept off. In fact, it was found that those whose HGH levels are high are able to lose almost 5 times the weight.

Muscle gain

An important rule of weight loss is that you have to replace the lost fast with lean muscle. These muscles are hardy and will not allow fat to be deposited in the body. Lean muscles can only be built by tearing into existing muscles. The torn muscle then starts reforming. The intermittent fast makes your body draw out all the fat and with regular exercise, you can easily kick start the process of developing lean muscles.

Insulin sensitivity

Insulin is a hormone that plays a vital role in the body. As discussed earlier, insulin helps to bind with the glucose present in the body and burns it to produce fuel. The intermittent fast controls the amount of glucose that is added to your body. This helps the insulin bind with the existing glucose stored as fat in your body and burn it to help you lose weight.

Visceral fat

One of your body's biggest enemies is visceral fat. This type of fat is extremely tough to get rid of and usually gathers around your waist, heart and other vital organs. With the help of intermittent fasting, it will be much easier for you to lose this type of fat. Fasting makes your body dig deep into the fat reserves and thus, slowly, but surely it will begin to melt the visceral fat away. By taking up an exercise routine to supplement the diet, you can further boost chances of losing this fat on a permanent basis.

Better immunity

It is no secret that your immune system has to be in top shape if you wish to lead a healthy life. Immunity is mostly controlled by the liver and gut. These organs are lined with cells that form the first line of defense against illnesses. If there is a lot of fat and toxins in your body then both the liver and gut will not work optimally. This can lead to compromised immunity. In such a case, it becomes important to cut down on the fat and toxins in the body. The intermittent fast helps in both regards. It helps in cutting into the fat and the consumption of liquids makes it easier to dissolve and eliminate the toxins from the body. This greatly improves immunity.

Free radicals

You must have heard of free radicals. These tend to react with molecules in your body and lead to oxidative damage. This can lead to many health issues and also inflammation. The intermittent fast helps bind these free radicals and controls the damage and inflammation to a large extent. This means you get to lead a fitter and more active life.

Lasting benefits

The intermittent fast ensures that you remain healthy, mentally and physically all through your life. It helps to cut down the risk associated with developing mental illnesses such as Alzheimer's and Parkinson's disease. These can be quite debilitating. Just by taking up the intermittent fast, you can cut down on the risk of developing these illnesses. A small step now can help you lead a healthier life when you grow old.

Longer life

With the amazing health benefits that the diet provides, it is obvious that you will lead a longer, healthier life. The intermittent fast is said to help you live a long life. Although there have been no conclusive studies on humans, one done on mice has revealed that it is possible to live up to 83% longer just by taking up the diet.

Weight loss

This list of benefits would be a little incomplete if we left out weight loss while listing out the benefits of the diet. Weight loss is possibly the biggest benefit associated with the diet. In fact, it is for this very reason that most people take up the diet. As per research, those who continue the diet religiously are able to lose about 8 to 9 pounds in about 2 months of starting the diet. The same research conducted a study on 300 people who were put on the diet for 4 months and found that those who took up the fast did not go through any significant loss in their appetites and yet lost quite a lot of weight. The intermittent fast is such that you will see better results if you are really fat. It is always the last few pounds that are difficult to lose. But remaining persistent will help you see positive results.

These are just some of the benefits associated with the fast and the benefits are not limited to these. As and when you take up intermittent fasting, you will start to reel in these benefits and more.

Chapter Seven: Seven Affordable Recipes to Minimize Calories

Omelette

Ingredients:

- 4 large eggs
- 1 tablespoon butter
- 1 large tomato, finely chopped
- 1 cup mushrooms, finely chopped
- 5 basil leaves, finely chopped
- 1 tablespoon parmesan cheese, grated
- 2 small pieces mozzarella
- 1 tablespoon green pesto
- Salt to taste
- Pepper to taste

Method:

- Add the eggs and water to a bowl and whisk until well combined.
- Add in the chopped mushrooms and tomatoes and mix until well combined.
- Add the salt and pepper and mix well.
- Add the butter to a pan and allow it to heat.
- Add the egg mixture on top and let the sides crisp-up.
- Flip it around to cook the other side. Avoid this if you want a runny yolk.
- Grate the mozzarella on top.
- Gently loosen it from the sides and add to a plate.
- Drizzle the pesto on top.
- Sprinkle the Parmesan and basil on top and serve.

Pork Chops

Ingredients:

- ½ cup olive oil
- 3 egg yolks, from large eggs
- 1 tablespoon lemon juice
- 3 pork loins with bones in, can also go for pork chops, about 1.7 ounces
- 2 tablespoons butter
- 3 ounces asparagus
- Salt to taste
- Pepper to taste

Method:

- To make the sauce, add the butter into a jar and microwave it to melt completely.
- Add in the egg yolks along with lemon juice and whizz until well combined.
- Go a little slow at the beginning and then pick up speed. Make sure the blender does not get too hot.
- Add in salt and pepper to taste.
- Place the frying pan over medium heat and melt the butter.
- Add the pork chops in and cook on each side for 6 to 7 minutes.
- In the meantime, add a pot to the stove and bring water to a boil.
- Add in the asparagus and allow it to blanch until soft. Drain it and add to a plate.
- Place the pork chops over the asparagus and drizzle the sauce on top.
- This can be served as both lunch and dinner.

Chicken meal

Ingredients:

- 1 tablespoon olive oil
- 1 onion, chopped
- 4 chicken thighs, skin removed
- 1 red bell pepper, cubed
- 1 yellow bell pepper, cubed
- 1 tablespoon corn flour
- 1.5 ounces yogurt, preferably fat free
- 1 tablespoon curry powder
- 2 garlic cloves, chopped
- 1 can tomatoes, chopped
- 3 tablespoons coriander leaves, roughly chopped
- Salt to taste
- Pepper to taste

Method:

- Add oil to a non-stick pan and place over medium heat.
- Toss in the onions and sauté it until brown or transparent.
- In the meantime, cut out any of the fat on the thigh of the chicken. Cut the thighs into 4 to 5 pieces and sprinkle salt and pepper on top and mix until well combined.
- Add the chicken to the pan along with the peppers and brown it on all sides. Move it around every few minutes.
- In the meantime, add the corn flour, water and yogurt to a bowl and mix until well combined.
- Add in the curry powder and the garlic and mix until well combined.
- Add in the tomatoes along with the yogurt mix and water and mix until well combined.
- Sprinkle the coriander on top.

- Allow the curry to simmer for about 30 minutes stirring the chicken every now and then.
- Sprinkle salt and pepper on top and serve hot.

Burger

Ingredients:

<u>Patties</u>

- 2 ounces ground beef
- 1 small garlic, chopped
- 1 small onion, chopped
- 1 teaspoon vinegar
- Salt to taste
- Pepper to taste
- 1 tablespoon oil

<u>Sauce</u>

- ¼ cup mayonnaise (home-made preferred)
- 2 tablespoons tomato puree or ketchup
- 1 tablespoon lemon juice
- Salt to taste
- Pepper to taste

<u>Burgers</u>

- Slider buns (whole wheat or any whole grain)
- 2 tablespoon butter
- 4 to 5 fresh lettuce leaves
- Pickles
- 1 medium onion, sliced
- 1 large tomato, sliced

Method:

- Slice through the center of the buns and place on a baking tray. Apply a mixture of egg yolk and water on top and place in a prebaked oven for 3 to 4 minutes or until the tops are crusty. You can also brown them on a pan with a little butter added in.
- Meanwhile, add the beef, chopped garlic, chopped onion, vinegar, salt and pepper to a bowl and mix until well combined. Do not over mix as that can lead to chewy and hard patties

- Make 4 or 5 small roundlets out of the mixture. Ensure they are smooth and do not have any cracks.
- Use a fork or knife to make holes in the patties.
- Rest the patties while you prepare the sauce.
- Add the mayo, tomato puree, pickle, salt and pepper and mix well.
- Add the butter to a hot pan and place the patties on top. Allow them to cook through completely. This should not take any more than 3 minutes.
- Once the patties are out, add in slices of bacon and cook them until completely crisp. They can also be crisped in the oven.
- To put the burger together, place the buns on a plate and apply the sauce on top.
- Add the patties in between and cover with a lettuce leaf.
- Add a piece of onion, tomato and pickles and cheese and cover with the other half.
- Place the burger under broiler and allow the cheese to melt completely.
- Serve hot.

Shrimp in Tomato Sauce

Ingredients:

- 1 tablespoons olive oil
- 2 garlic cloves, chopped
- 1 red chili, flaked and chopped
- 2 large tomatoes, chopped
- 1 large lemon, freshly squeezed
- 8 ounces large prawns
- 3 tablespoons parsley
- Salt to taste
- Pepper to taste
- 2 cups green beans, steamed

Method:

- Add the oil to a pan and keep on low heat.
- Toss in the garlic and chilli and cook until the garlic goes brown. Keep stirring so that it does not over brown.
- Toss in the tomatoes and lemon juice and mix until well combined.
- The tomatoes have to soften up completely.
- Add in the prawns and mix well.
- Remember never to overcook the prawns as that can make them go solid.
- Remove the prawns from the heat and add to a plate.
- Serve with a sprinkling of pepper and the beans on top.

Pepper Beef

Ingredients:

- 2 thick cut steaks, fat removed
- ½ cup yogurt, fat free
- ½ teaspoon horseradish
- 1 garlic clove, minced
- ½ bowl salad leaves
- 1 cup button mushrooms
- 1 large red onion, chopped
- 1 teaspoon olive oil
- Salt to taste
- Pepper to taste

Method:

- Add the steaks to a pan along with the pepper and salt and rub until well combined.
- Add the yogurt, horseradish, garlic, salt and pepper to a bowl and mix until well combined.
- Toss in the salad leaves along with the mushrooms and mix well.
- Add the onions and mix gently.
- Add the oil to the pan and heat gently.
- Add the steaks and cook it over high heat for a couple of minutes.
- Turn it around until it is browned on all sides.
- It is best to cook it until medium rare for 4 minutes or can go for well done for 5 minutes.
- Add the steak to a plate and rest it for a few minutes.
- Add the salad leaves on the plate and place thinly sliced steak on top of it.
- Sprinkle onions on top and serve hot.

Stir-fried Pork

Ingredients:

- 10 ounces pork tenderloin, fat cut out
- 1 teaspoon corn flour
- 2 tablespoons soya sauce
- 1 tablespoon olive oil
- 2 cups button mushrooms, chopped
- 2 red peppers, chopped
- 2-inch ginger piece
- 1 garlic, chopped
- 4 spring onions, chopped
- Salt to taste
- Pepper to taste

Method:

- Add the pork to a bowl along with the salt and pepper and mix until well combined.
- Add in water and soy and mix well.
- Add the oil to a pan and place on medium heat.
- Add the pork to it and stir fry it for 2 minutes or until it is browned evenly but not completely cooked through.
- Add it to a plate.
- Add the pan back to the heat and reduce the heat and add in some more oil to it.
- Toss in the mushrooms and pepper and mix for 2 to 3 minutes.
- Toss on the garlic and ginger along with the onions and mix until well combined.
- Add the pork to the pan and pour the sauce over it.
- Cook it for about 5 minutes or until the sauce has thickened and serve hot.

These recipes are simple and can be made within 30 minutes. But do not limit yourself to just these and experiment with new recipes.

Chapter Eight: The 21-day Intermittent Fasting Weight Loss Ritual

Here is a 21-day fasting ritual to follow for weight loss.

Day 1: Start your day with breakfast at 12 noon. Go for an omelette and banana milkshake. Have your lunch by 4 p.m., go for a vegetable burger and finish off dinner by having bowl of salad. Eat your dinner by 8 p.m. For morning snack go for fat-free yogurt with mixed fruit.

Day 2: Start your day with a simple pancake. Supplement it with a tall glass of orange juice. For lunch, go for wheat based flatbread and mutton gravy. For dinner, consume any leftover flatbreads and curry. Munch on mixed nuts for your snack.

Day 3: For breakfast, choose poached eggs with asparagus spears. For lunch, go for the pork stir-fry mentioned in the recipe section of this book. For dinner, go for a turkey salad. It is a good time to stop your snacks at this point, as your body will be getting accustomed to the new eating schedule.

Day 4: For breakfast, choose waffles with mixed berries and a honey drizzle. For lunch, go for the shrimp dish mentioned in the recipe section of this book. For dinner, go for a bowl of fresh fruit with yogurt drizzled on top. At this point, you have to incorporate a light exercise routine. Go for a simple cardio-based workout.

Day 5: For breakfast, choose boiled eggs with a simple salad. For lunch go for wild rice with Thai green curry. Go for steamed fish with ginger for dinner. At this point, move your dinner timing back by an hour and have it by 7 p.m.

Day 6: For breakfast, go for the omelette mentioned in the recipe section of this book and supplement it with a glass of strawberry smoothie. For lunch, go for sweet potato salad. For dinner, have a steak of your choice. Continue the exercise routine and add a different workout like cross fit.

Day 7: for breakfast go for spinach in omelette. For lunch go for the beef dish mentioned in the recipe section of this book. For dinner, consume any leftover beef and supplement it with an easy salad. Take stock of the week and everything that you ate. Make a note of it and keep track of your progress.

Day 8: For breakfast go for chicken tortillas. For lunch, choose grilled fish in butter sauce. As for dinner, go for mushroom soup. At this point, it is best to move your breakfast timing ahead by an hour. Push it to 1 p.m. So, your new meal timings will be 1 p.m. breakfast, 4 p.m. lunch and 7 p.m. dinner.

Day 9: For breakfast go for Moroccan chicken skewers. For lunch, go for the burger mentioned in the recipe section of this book. For dinner, go for chicken soup with whole wheat bread. Increase your exercise timing by about 30 minutes. Focus on areas that need the most work.

Day 10: For breakfast, have oatmeal with a selection of cut fruit. For lunch, choose salmon with veggies. For dinner, go for chili bean bowl. Make sure you have plenty of fluids during the fasting periods.

Day 11: For breakfast, go for a mixed bean salad with a glass of orange juice. For dinner, go for roasted vegetables with steak of your choice. As you can see, it is time to eliminate one meal from your diet. It is best to start by removing the middle meal as that way your body will not be too stressed.

Day 12: For breakfast go for tofu wraps. For dinner, choose cauliflower rice with mixed vegetables and bean curry. Make sure you do not stop exercising. Add in a new routine such as swimming or dancing.

Day 13: For breakfast, go for mixed vegetable quinoa and a glass of mango smoothie. For dinner, choose chicken Panzanella salad. At this point, move your dinner timing back by an hour. So, if you have dinner by 7 p.m., move it back to 6 p.m. Keep up the exercise routine.

Day 14: For breakfast, go for deviled eggs with a large avocado. For dinner, choose the chicken meal mentioned in the recipe section of this book. At the end of week 2, look back at the week and make a note of all the changes you have experienced.

Day 15: For breakfast, go for cereal with mixed fruit and a glass of pineapple smoothie. For dinner, go for chicken salad with mixed greens. You can move your breakfast ahead by one hour. Move it to 2 p.m. This means that you eat your two meals within a 4-hour window. Keep up with the exercise routine.

Day 16: For breakfast, go for the omelette mentioned in the recipe section of this book and a glass of lemongrass tea. For dinner, choose the pork stir fry mentioned in the recipe section of this book.

Day 17: For breakfast, go for hard-boiled eggs and a glass of banana milkshake. For dinner, go for the beef dish mentioned in the recipe section of this book. Keep meals simple and clean. Make sure you buy quality ingredients from organic markets.

Day 18: For breakfast, go for mixed vegetable quinoa and a glass of ginger ale for dinner, go for chicken sandwich.

Day 19: For breakfast, have chicken salad. For dinner, go for the shrimp dish mentioned in the recipe section of this book. Keep up the exercise routine and push yourself harder.

Day 20: For breakfast, go for spinach omelette and a glass of watermelon juice. For dinner, have poached salmon with butter sauce.

Day 21: For breakfast, go for grilled tofu and a glass of mango smoothie. For dinner, choose the pork chops mentioned in the recipe section of this book.

This is a simple 21-day intermittent schedule that you can follow. However, you can make modifications to suit your needs. Feel free to mix up the dishes. You must persist with the exercise routine.

Chapter Nine: Motivation for you While Intermittent Fasting

It is understood that it is not always easy to stay on a diet. Although the intermittent fast cannot be thought of as a diet, it requires you to make lifestyle and food choices that can be a little taxing at times.

In this chapter, we will look at simple things that you can do to stick with the fast.

Expectations

It is obvious that you will have a lot of expectations from the diet. It is normal to have them, as you will want to reach your ideal weight within a certain period of time. But what is important to note is that you have to have realistic expectations when it comes to the time frame you set to achieve the weight loss. You cannot achieve it overnight. If you are obese now, then try to go for a 6 to 12-month plan to lose weight. If you go for something lesser then it might not work out for you. If you set an unrealistic goal and see that it is not working out for you then you will feel discouraged and might want to go off the diet. It is therefore important to set realistic goals in order to achieve them better.

Motivators

Make sure you know exactly why you are going for the weight loss routine. It is obvious that you will want to lose weight and fit into smaller clothes etc. But apart from these, there have to be other motivators as well that will keep you on track. Make a list of them and stick them in your room or have a copy of the list on your phone so that you can look at it and remain motivated. These will keep you from going for something unhealthy and sticking with the fast.

Clear out the kitchen

A top tip is to get rid of all junk and processed foods from the kitchen. These can be quite tempting. Follow the rule, "out of sight, out of mind." Go through everything in the kitchen and get rid of all items that are bad for the diet. Keep it off the shelves and off the counters. Replace them with healthier alternatives such as nuts. Make sure you do not go into the kitchen after a certain point in time say 10 or 11 at night. Once you have had your last meal, stay away from the kitchen area. If you have a lot of junk and processed food lying around then throw a party to finish it all in one go.

Don't be too harsh

Don't be too harsh on yourself if you end up going for a cheat meal. It can be a little difficult to make a sudden change in your lifestyle. It is therefore advisable to go slow with it. Make sure you ease into the diet so that you can stave off temptations. Do not be tempted to fall off the wagon just because you had one cheat meal. Treat it as a cheat and focus on your fast.

Carry your food

Do not forget to carry your meals everywhere you go. Be it to the office or to a party, you have to carry the meals with you so that you can avoid the hassle of settling for something that is forbidden by the diet. If you don't have a ready snack with you then you are bound to go for something unhealthy. Have a high-protein snack ready that you can bite into as soon as you get hungry. A few good options include peanuts, almonds and a hard-boiled egg. These can keep you going until the next meal.

Don't go for too much

If you are just starting out with the fast then make sure you go slowly. Do not do too many things at once, as that will confuse your body. If you do not exercise at all then go for simple ones at first. Once you have settled into the diet, go for an exercise routine. If you start both at once then you will do justice to neither. But make sure at some point you take up exercising and do not rely on the fast alone. It would be best to wait for about a month before taking up an exercise regime. Although research suggests you have to stick to something for at least a month for the habit to stick, it is best you take it up seriously and continue for at least 6 months to a year.

Do your research

It is obvious that in this day and age nobody can go without eating out. It can be quite a challenge to go out and not find something edible on the menu. In such a case, it pays to do your research and make sure you find a restaurant that serves meals that cater to your choice. It will be even better if you find something that customizes the menu for you. If you are traveling, then plan ahead and find out which places you can eat at. Pack enough food to keep you going for at least 3 days. Make sure you go for foods that can last at least a week.

Reward yourself

It is always important to reward yourself with something nice for keeping up the good work. It can be a trip to the spa or a vacation. You can also buy yourself something that you have always wanted like a crock-pot or an air fryer. A recipe book too can serve as a reward. The reward can be anything as long as you feel motivated to keep up with the diet. It would be advisable not to go for a cheat meal as a reward.

Mindfulness and meditation

Mindfulness is a technique that helps you dig deep into your thoughts and remain completely focused on the task at hand. By practicing mindful eating, you give yourself the chance to enjoy a healthy meal. Those who enjoy their meals are able to better connect with the food and lose a significant amount of weight just by remaining focused on the meal. Another research found that mindfulness successfully put an end to binge eating. It is said to have reduced from almost 4 to 1.5 times a week over a period of 6 weeks. It is, therefore, a good idea to indulge in mindfulness eating. You can also engage in meditation. This can keep your mind calm. Try to stay away from stress as much as possible as it can negatively impact your health. It can also cause you to gain weight. The more stress free you remain, the better off you are in terms of attaining weight loss.

Keep track

Keep track of your progress. This can serve as a big motivator to keep you on track. Maintain a diary and write down everything including your weight, measurements, meal timings, meal plans, etc. Refer back to it from time to time to ensure that you are on the right track. It is a good idea to maintain a blog and keep updating your progress. Your friends and family members can access it and encourage you to keep up the good work.

Partner up

Getting a partner is always a great way to remain motivated to stick to a fast. Not only will you have company, you will also remain motivated to keep t it. It can be a spouse, partner, sibling, colleague, friend, etc., as long as they wish to benefit from the fast. Usually, when one partner decides to make a healthy choice be it dietary modification or exercise, the other decides to follow as well. You will also find it easier with your partner chipping in to prepare the healthy meals and keeping track of your progress.

Go for a heavy breakfast

There is nothing better than a healthy and hearty breakfast or rather the first meal of the day. If you plan on having your meal by 12 noon then go for something that is loaded with proteins and other nutrients. As per studies, women who ate 1.05 ounces of protein for breakfast were able to avoid feeling peckish before lunch as compared to those who ate a breakfast low in proteins. You can also have a protein and fiber rich lunch to supplement the breakfast.

Take your time

Don't be in a hurry to get through everything at once. Go about it in a slow and steady manner. As mentioned earlier, it might take at least a month for you to make a habit stick. Be patient with it. Keep at it for at least 6 months. Do not compare yourself to others. If there are people passing negative comments, then learn to ignore them. You have to remain focused and motivated to achieve the slimmer, fitter and better you.

Customize

Customize the diet for yourself. Only you will know your body best. Do not follow what someone else is following as what works for them might not work for you. It is best to come up with a plan that is sustainable in the long run as compared to one that will only provide you momentary results.

These are just some of the things you can do to remain motivated. Do not limit it to just these and do whatever it takes for you to stick with the intermittent fast.

Conclusion

I thank you once again for choosing this book and hope you had a good time reading it. The main aim of this book was to educate you on the basics of the intermittent fast and how you can use it to lose excess weight and develop a strong and healthy body.

The intermittent fast is sure to help you attain your ideal body weight. This is especially useful for those who are trying to get rid of excess weight and keep it from coming back on. Apart from shedding weight, you will also benefit greatly from the positive health effects that the diet provides.

But remember that you will only be able to sustain the results if you put in hard work and dedication. Do not assume that you will remain with the results forever just by adopting the diet. Keep at it if you want to maintain it.

As mentioned in the book, you have to make sure that you know what works well for your body as everybody has different needs. You might have to engage in a little trial and error to come up with a strategy that works best for you. Make sure you stick with the strategy and allow it to modify your life.

Here is a summary of the things we read in the book.

- The 16/8 diet where you fast for 16 hours and consume meals within the next 8-hour window
- The 5:2 diet where you have your regular meals 5 days a week and fast on 2 days
- The 24-hour fast where you do not eat anything for 24 hours. As discussed, this can be a little extreme but can provide lasting results
- Alternate day fasting is where you do not eat every alternate day. This too might sound quite extreme but will get a little easier as you go. Make sure your body and mind are fully prepared for it before taking it up

Remember that it is always best to err on the side of caution; consult your physician before taking on any of the intermittent fast. It is especially important if you suffer from conditions such as diabetes, hypoglycemia, heart disease and other such illnesses.

I wish you luck with your weight loss endeavors and hope you see positive results at the earliest. But do not limit your knowledge to this book alone and read as much as you can on the topic.

References:

https://www.healthline.com/nutrition/intermittent-fasting-guide

https://www.healthline.com/nutrition/what-is-intermittent-fasting

https://www.mindbodygreen.com/articles/intermittent-fasting-diet-plan-how-to-schedule-meals

https://www.getthegloss.com/article/the-5-2-diet-plan-week-one

https://www.foodnetwork.com/healthyeats/healthy-tips/2013/07/the-health-benefits-of-berries

https://www.ncbi.nlm.nih.gov/pmc/articles/PMC4733124/

https://www.newsweek.com/high-energy-breakfast-weight-loss-type-2-diabetes-852028

About The Author

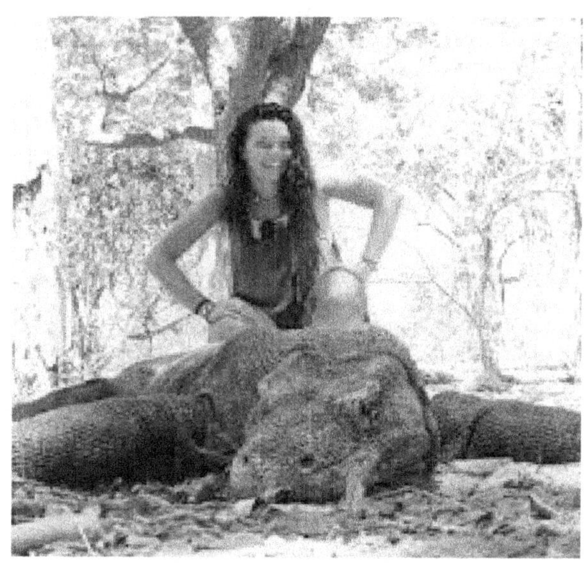

Debra Litchfield is an avid traveler, animal lover, passionate dietitian, and weight loss coach. She has been helping her clients reach their weight loss and diet goals for just over 10 years with great success. Today, Debra still coaches on occasion but prefers to shares her teachings through books and audio. This way she can travel and do what she loves while still helping others reach their weight loss goals!

Don't forget your Free Book!

As a token of appreciation for you purchasing my book, I would like to throw in a **free book!**

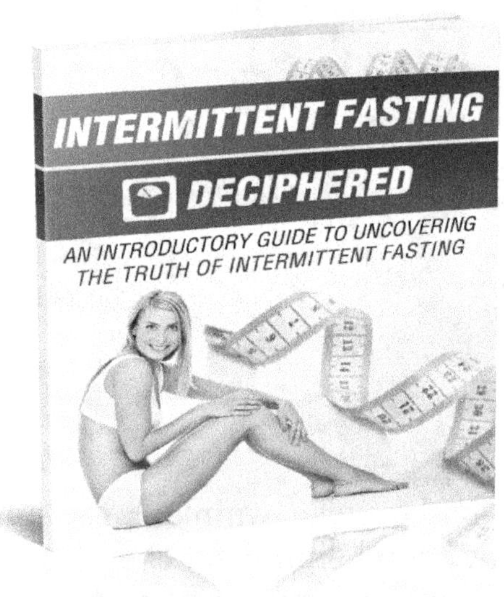

Click Here For Your Free e-Book!

In addition to receiving your free book you will also be able to receive free weight loss and diet advice, have a chance to review my books before they come out, and much more!

www.ingramcontent.com/pod-product-compliance
Lightning Source LLC
Chambersburg PA
CBHW081635250726
48657CB00009B/2887